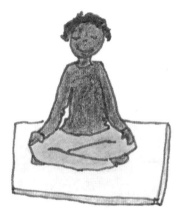

MINDFUL MOVEMENTS

A portion of the proceeds of
every book sold goes to support
nonprofit projects in Vietnam.

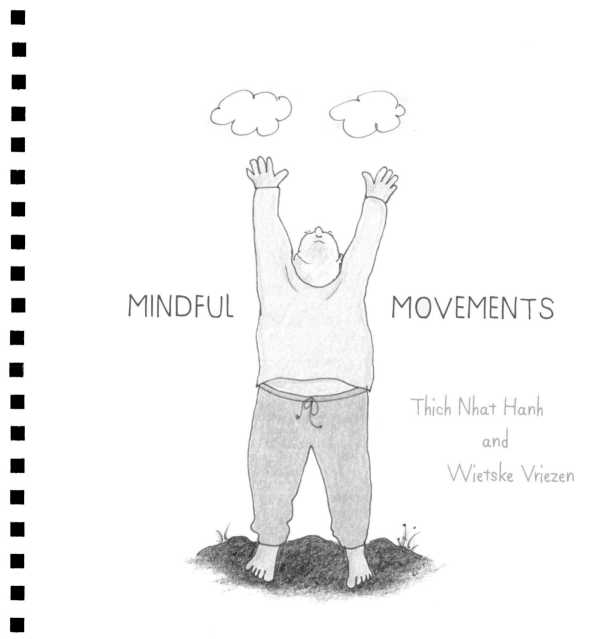

MINDFUL MOVEMENTS

Thich Nhat Hanh
and
Wietske Vriezen

Parallax Press
P.O. Box 7355
Berkeley, California 94707
www.parallax.org

Parallax Press is the publishing division of
Unified Buddhist Church, Inc.
© 2008 by Unified Buddhist Church.
All rights reserved.
Printed in China.

Cover and text design by Debbie Berne, Herter Studio LLC.
Cover and interior illustrations by Wietske Vriezen.
Parallax Press would like to thank Sounds True for giving permission to
include the DVD in this book.
The publisher would also like to thank Melanie Green.

Library of Congress Cataloging-in-Publication Data
Nhat Hanh, Thich.
Mindful movements : mindfulness exercises developed by Thich Nhat Hanh
and the Plum Village Sangha / Thich Nhat Hanh and Wietske Vriezen.
    p. cm.
ISBN 978-1-888375-79-4
1. Meditation—Buddhism. 2. Spiritual life—Buddhism. I. Vriezen, Wietske.
II. Title.
 BQ9800.T5392N4546 2008
 294.3'4435—dc22
                 2007044759

7 8 9 / 16 15 14

TABLE OF CONTENTS

INTRODUCTION

MINDFULNESS is our ability to be aware of what is going on both inside us and around us. It is the continuous awareness of our bodies, emotions, and thoughts. Through mindfulness, we avoid harming ourselves and others, and we can work wonders. If we live mindfully in everyday life, walk mindfully, are full of love and caring, then we create a miracle and transform the world into a wonderful place.

The object of your mindfulness can be anything. You can look at the sky and breathe in and say, "Breathing in, I'm aware of the blue sky." So you are mindful of the blue sky. The blue sky becomes the object of your mindfulness. "Breathing out, I smile to the blue sky." Smiling is another kind of practice. First of all, you recognize the blue sky as existing. And if you continue the practice, you will see that the blue sky is wonderful. It may be that you've lived thirty or forty years but you have never seen and touched the blue sky that deeply.

In the Sutra on the Four Establishments of Mindfulness, the Buddha offers four layers of mindfulness practice: mindfulness of the body, of the emotions, of the mind, and of the objects of mind. Practicing mindfulness at each layer can be the foundation of well-being and happiness. When we don't practice mindfulness, we suffer in our body, our mind, and in our relationships. In practicing mindfulness, we become a peaceful refuge for ourselves and others. When the seed of mindfulness in us is watered, it can grow into enlightenment, understanding, compassion, and transformation. The more we practice mindfulness, the stronger this seed will grow.

Clarity flows from mindfulness. When we are mindful, we can practice Right Thinking and Right Speech. With the energy of mindfulness, we can always return to our true home, the present moment.

The Chinese character for mindfulness reveals its meaning. The upper part of the character means "now" and the lower part stands for "mind" or "heart." The Vietnamese word for mindfulness, *chan niem,* means to be truly in the present moment. Mindfulness helps us to come back to the here and now, to be aware of what is going on in the present moment, and to be in touch with the wonders of life.

THE SEVEN MIRACLES OF MINDFULNESS

If we bring mindfulness into every aspect of our life, we cannot help but experience life's miracles.

THE FIRST MIRACLE is to be present and able to touch deeply the miracles of life, like the blue sky, a flower, the smile of a child.

THE SECOND MIRACLE is to make the other—the sky, a flower, a child—present also. Then we have the opportunity to see each other deeply.

THE THIRD MIRACLE is to nourish the object of your attention with full awareness and appropriate attention.

THE FOURTH MIRACLE is to relieve the suffering of others.

THE FIFTH MIRACLE is looking deeply into the nature of self and others.

THE SIXTH MIRACLE is understanding. If we are mindful of the present moment, we can see deeply and things become clear. With understanding, the desire to relieve suffering and give love will awaken within us.

THE SEVENTH MIRACLE is transformation. By practicing Right Mindfulness, we touch the healing and refreshing aspects of life and begin to transform the suffering in ourselves and in the world.

Our true home is the present moment. If we really live in the moment, our worries and hardships will disappear and we will discover life with all its miracles. Real life can only be found and touched in the here and now. This is because the present moment is the only moment we can actually experience and influence. The past is over and the future has not yet arrived. Since the present moment is the only real moment for us, we can always return here to get in touch with the wonders of life.

As long as we are consumed with our everyday problems—distress about the present, regrets about the past, or constant worries about the future—we cannot be free people; we are not able to live in the here and now.

BREATHING AND MOVING MINDFULLY

No one can be successful in the art of meditation without having passed through the gate of breathing. The practice of mindfulness encompasses all spheres and activities, including ordinary actions and our every breath.

We often assume breathing is just a natural skill; everyone knows how to inhale and exhale. But breathing is a miracle. Being aware of our breath not only helps us manage the difficulties in everyday life, it also helps develop our wisdom and compassion. We can sit and breathe, but it is just as important to practice mindful breathing while we are moving.

Life is a path, but life is not about getting to a certain place. The Mindful Movements and walking meditation are ways to practice moving without a goal or intention. Mindful walking simply means walking while being aware of each step and of our breath. It can be practiced anywhere, whether you are alone in nature or with others in a crowded city. You can even practice mindful breathing and walking meditation in between business appointments or in the parking lot of the supermarket. Walking on this planet is a joy. Mindful walking allows us to be aware of the pleasure of walking. We can keep our steps slow, relaxed, and calm. There is no rush, no place to get to, no hurry. Mindful walking can release our sorrows and our worries and help bring peace into our body and mind.

We can practice walking meditation alone, with another person, or with a group. Placing our footsteps one after the other slowly and in silence, we can create joy with each step. If we take steps without anxiety, in peace and joy, then we will cause a flower to bloom on the earth with every step.

THE TEN MINDFUL MOVEMENTS are another wonderful way of connecting your mind and body in mindfulness. They are a way to touch the sky, to smile at your own body, and to touch your heart. When you do them, please enjoy each part of each movement. Do what you can. They are not like aerobics, where you have to move as quickly as possible. There is no need to rush. When I do them, I find I cannot help smiling. I hope they bring you joy.

Thich Nhat Hanh

THE TEN MINDFUL MOVEMENTS

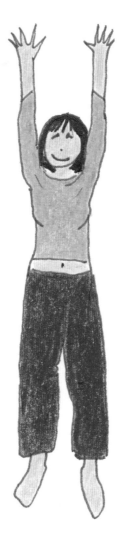

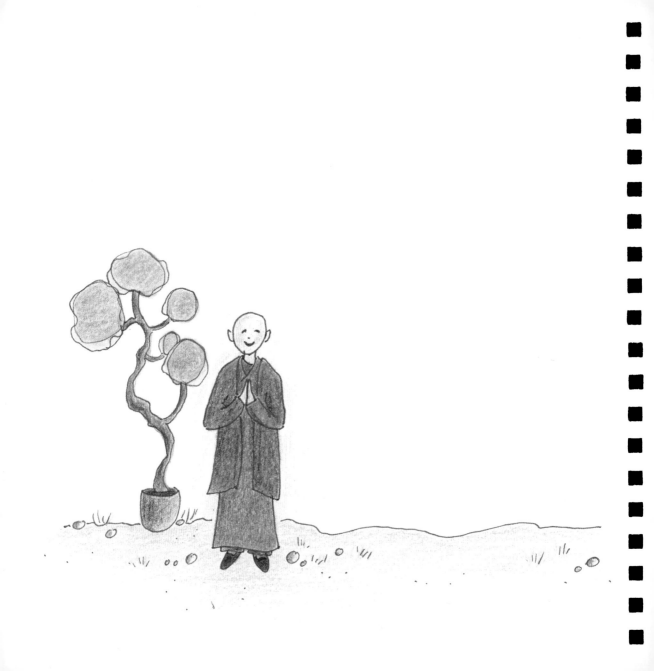

This is Thich Nhat Hanh. His friends call him "Thay."

He's a Vietnamese Buddhist monk.

Thich Nhat Hanh grew up in Vietnam at a time
when there was a lot of conflict and violence.
He was exiled because of his outspoken peace activities
during the Vietnam War. Thich Nhat Hanh saw that it
was very important for each person to practice finding
peace within themselves. So in 1982, he founded Plum
Village, a community of monks, nuns, laymen,
and laywomen in southwest France.

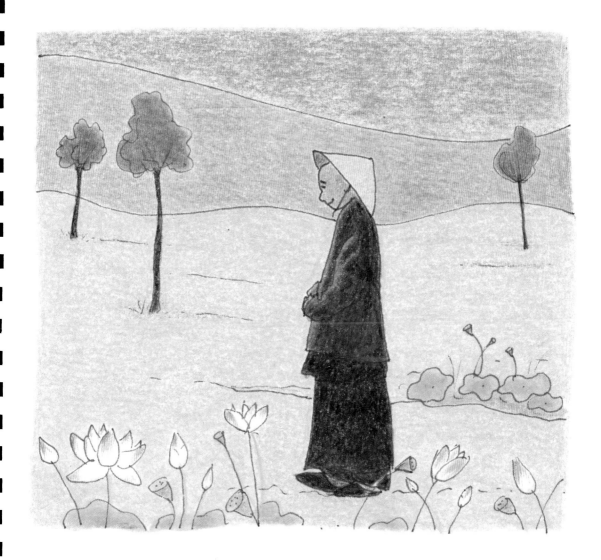

When people have peace in themselves,

then there can be peace in the world.

This is our practice every day.

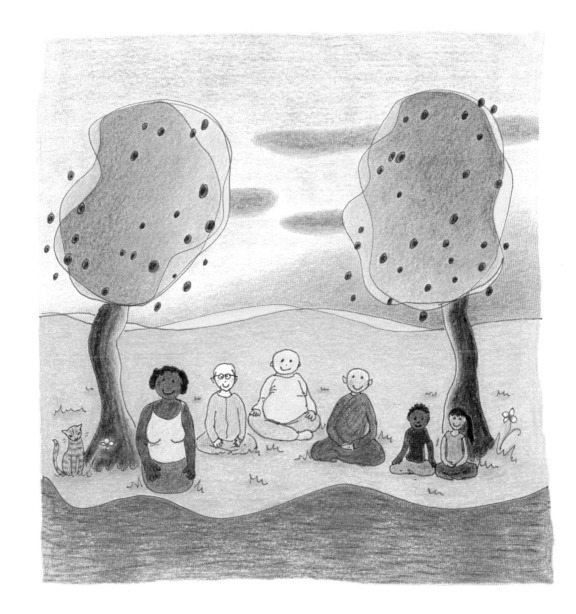

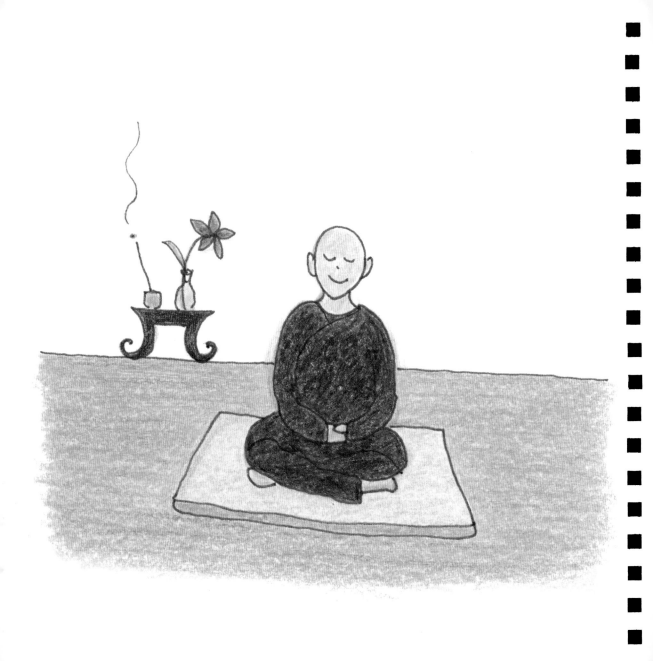

One way people can develop peace in themselves

is by just sitting quietly and breathing.

This is called meditation.

With each in-breath, we can notice we are
breathing in. With each out-breath, we can notice
we are breathing out. When we breathe like this,
our body and our mind come together. And when our
body and our mind are together, we are capable of living
life more fully. We are able to enjoy what is going
on in and around us in each moment.

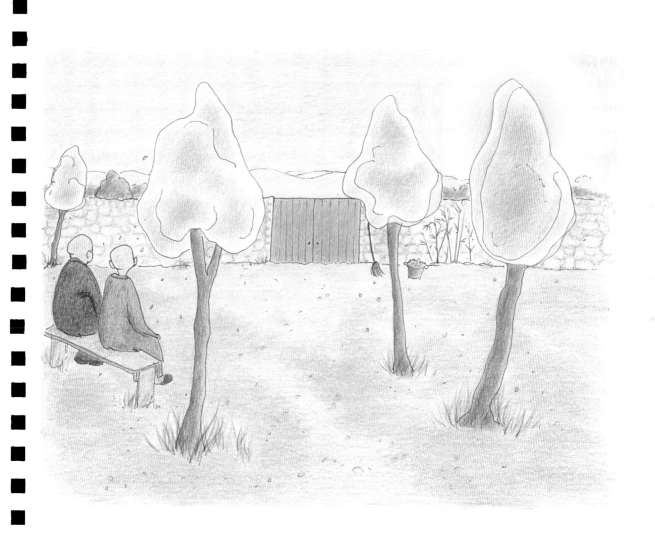

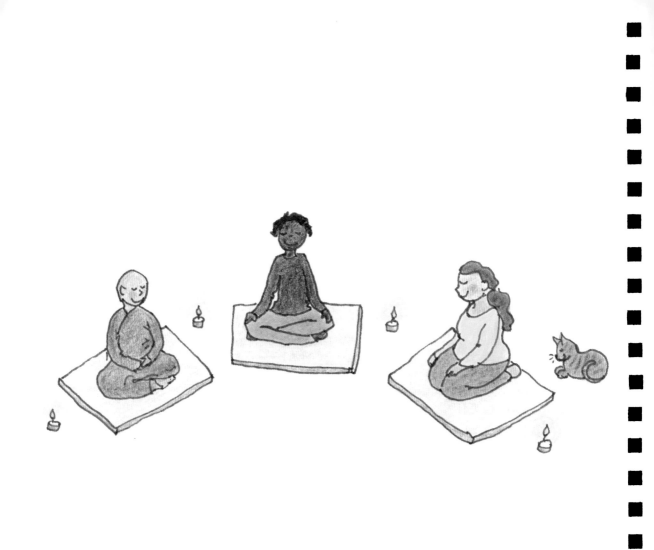

Often it helps to meditate with other people.
Sitting together, breathing together, we
can feel very peaceful and happy.

But sometimes we need to stop sitting in one place
and start to move around! Thich Nhat Hanh has developed
exercises called the Ten Mindful Movements. The practice
of the Mindful Movements is to bring awareness and
enjoyment into our bodies and into the movements we
make with our bodies. Mindful Movements are very simple
but very deep. They have been taught and practiced in
Plum Village for over two decades.

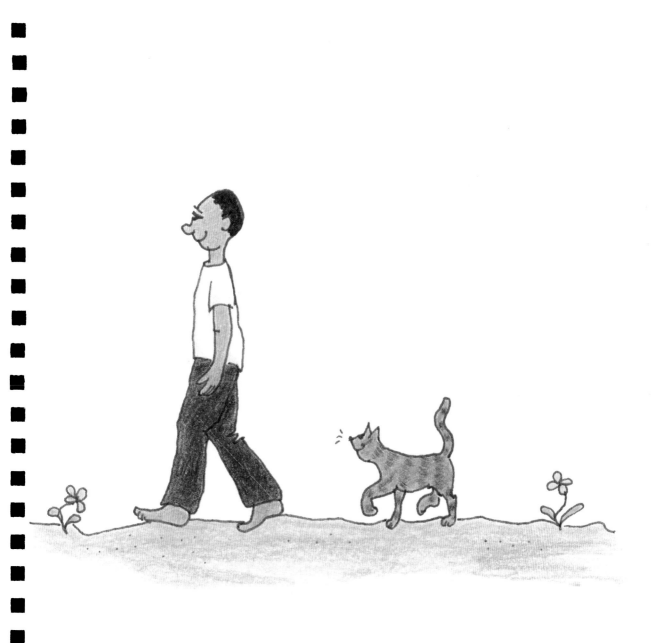

The exercises are easy to do at home, by yourself, or with others. You can do them inside or outside in the park. You can do them every day or just once in a while. Do each movement four times before moving on to the next one. Have fun!

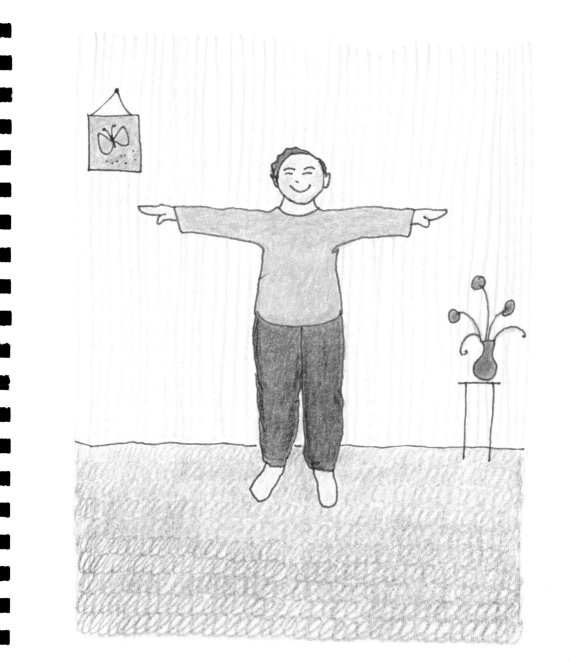

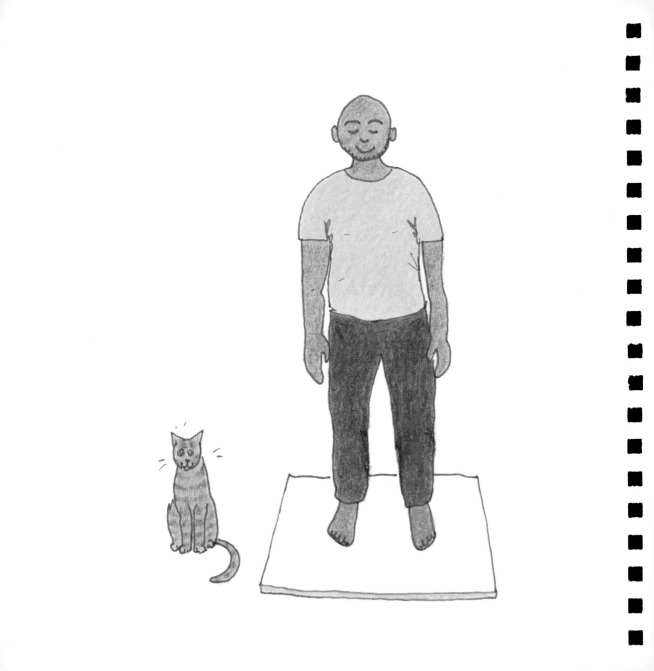

To begin, stand with your feet firmly on the ground, shoulder-width apart. Your knees are soft, slightly bent and not locked. Stand upright and relaxed. Your shoulders are loose. Imagine an invisible thread is attached to the top of your head and it pulls you up toward the sky. Keeping your body straight, tuck your chin in slightly so your neck can relax.

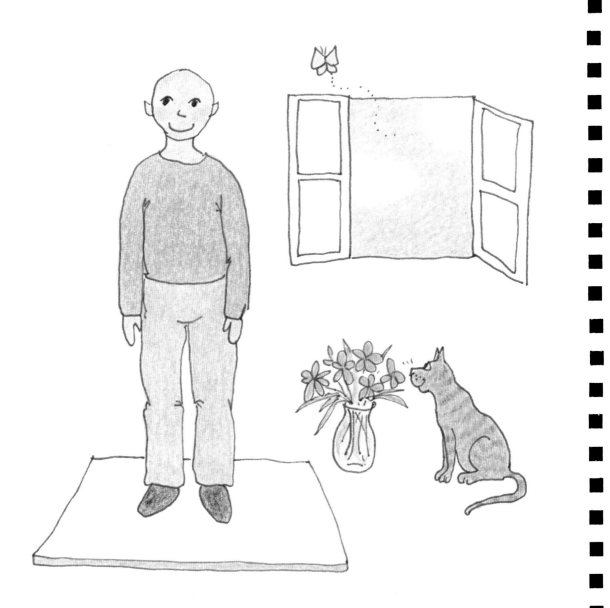

Let's practice a little bit of conscious breathing.
Make sure your feet are placed firmly on the earth,
your body is centered and your back is straight.
Allow your in-breath to come down into your belly.
Then exhale completely. Continue to breathe slowly,
aware of each in-breath and out-breath. Smile and
enjoy standing like this for a moment.

MINDFUL MOVEMENT #1

Begin with your feet slightly apart, arms at your sides.

Breathing in, keep your elbows straight as you lift

your arms in front of you until they're shoulder level,

horizontal to the ground. Breathing out, bring

your arms down again to your sides.

Repeat the movement three more times.

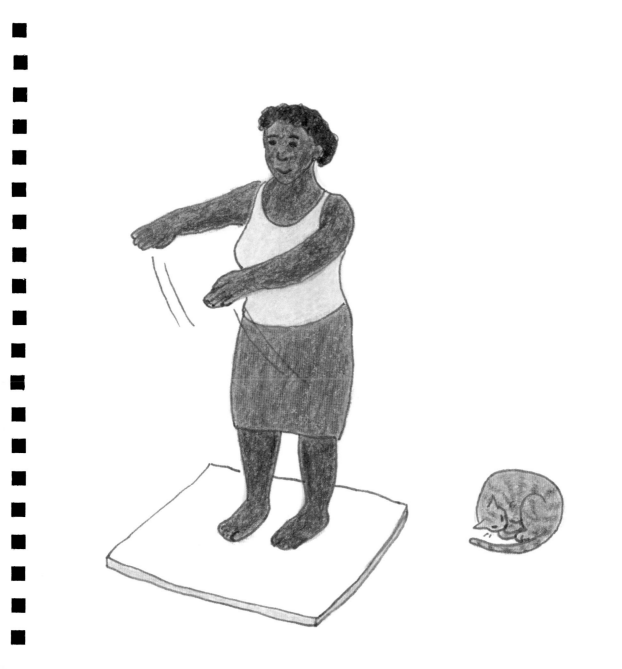

MINDFUL MOVEMENT #2

Begin with your arms at your sides. Breathing in, lift your arms in front of you. In one continuous movement, bring them all the way up, stretching them above your head. Touch the sky! This movement can be done with your palms either facing inward toward each other, or facing forward as you reach up. Breathing out, bring your arms slowly down again to your sides.

Repeat three more times.

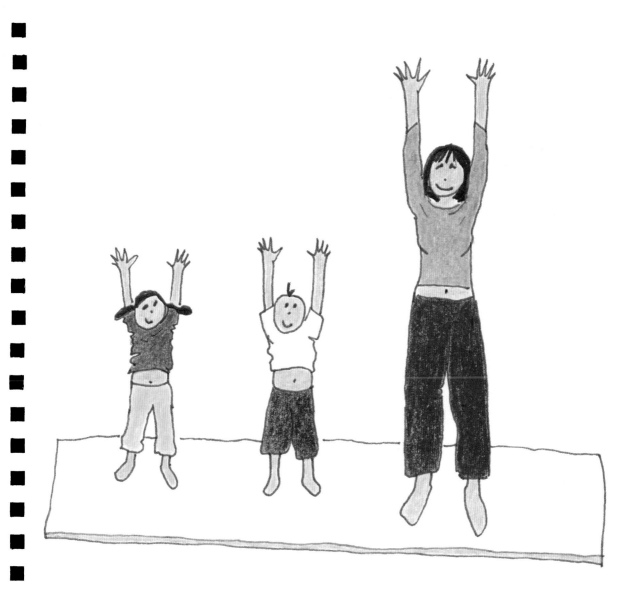

Breathing in, lift your arms out to the side, palms up, until your arms are shoulder level, parallel to the ground. Breathing out, touch your shoulders with your fingertips, keeping your upper arms horizontal. Breathing in, open your arms, extending them until they're stretched out to a horizontal position again. Breathing out, bend your elbows, bringing your fingertips back to your shoulders.

When you breathe in, you are like a flower opening to the warm sun. Breathing out, the flower closes. From this position with your fingertips on your shoulders, do the movement three more times. Then lower your arms back down to your sides.

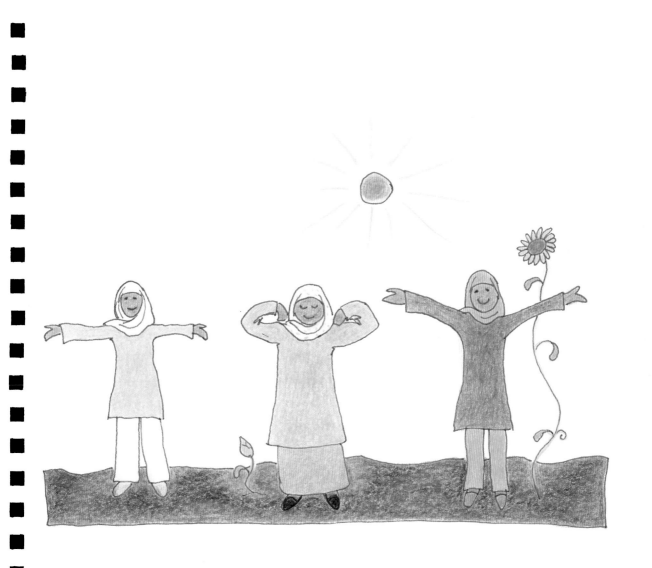

MINDFUL MOVEMENT #4

In this exercise, you make a large circle with your arms.
Breathing in, bring your arms straight down in front
of you, centered between your hips, palms together.
Raise your arms up and separate your hands so your
arms can stretch up over your head. Breathing out,
continue the circle, arms circling back, until your fingers
point toward the ground. Breathing in, lift your arms back
and reverse the circle. Breathe out as you bring
your palms together and your arms come down in
front of you. Repeat three more times.

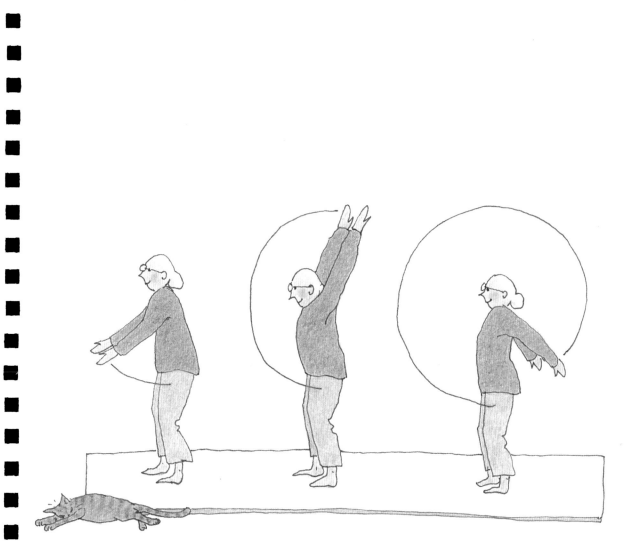

Start by putting your hands on your waist.

As you do this exercise, keep your legs straight but not locked, and your head centered over your body. Breathing in, bend forward at the waist and begin to make a circle with your upper body. When you're halfway through the circle, your upper body leaning back, breathe out and complete the circle, ending with your head in front of you while you're still bent at the waist. On your next in-breath, begin a circle in the opposite direction. On your out-breath, complete the circle. Repeat the series of movements three more times.

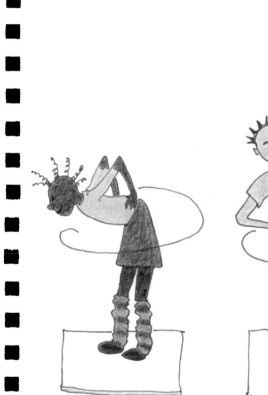
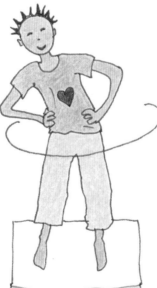
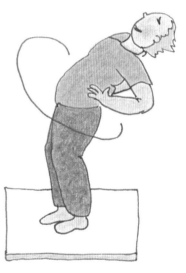

MINDFUL MOVEMENT #6

This exercise is called The Frog.

Begin with your hands on your waist, heels together, feet turned out to form a V, so that they make a 90° angle. Breathing in, rise up on your toes. Breathing out, stay on your toes, keep your back straight, and bend your knees. Keeping your upper body centered, go down as low as you comfortably can maintaining your balance. Breathing in, straighten your knees and come all the way up, still standing on your toes. From this position, repeat the movement three more times, remembering to breathe slowly and deeply.

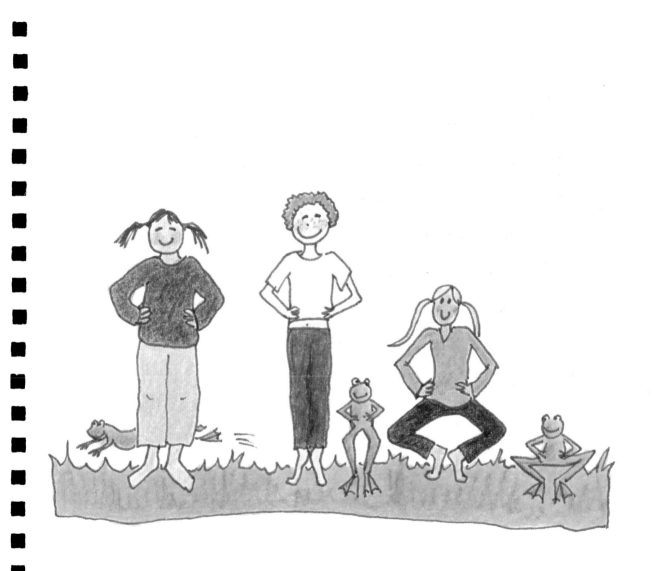

MINDFUL MOVEMENT #7

In this exercise, you touch the sky and the earth.

Your feet are hip-width apart. Breathing in,

bring your arms up above your head, palms forward.

Stretch all the way up, and look up as you touch the sky.

Breathing out, bend at the waist as you bring your arms

down to touch the earth. Release your neck. From this

position, breathe in, and keep your back straight as you

come all the way back up and touch the sky.

Touch the earth and sky three more times.

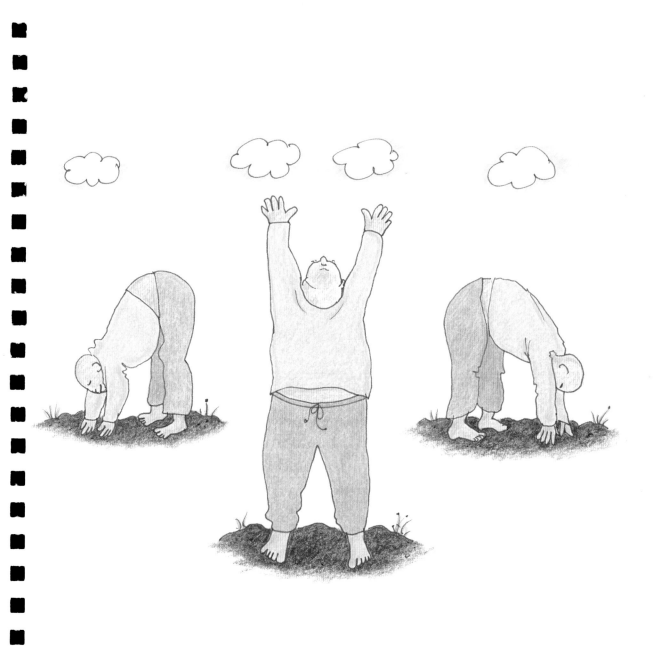

MINDFUL MOVEMENT #8

Start with your feet together and your hands on your waist. Begin by putting all your weight on to your left foot. Breathing in, lift your right thigh as you bend your knee and keep your toes pointed toward the ground. Breathing out, stretch your right leg out in front of you, keeping your toes pointed. Breathing in, bend your knee and bring your foot back toward your body. Breathing out, put your right foot back on the ground. Next put all your weight on to your right foot and do the movement with the other leg. Repeat the series of movements three more times.

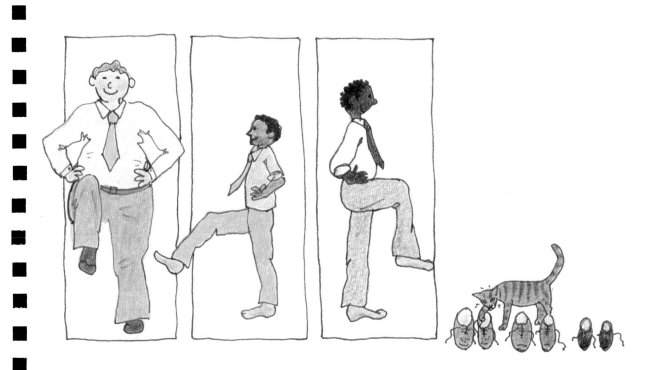

In this exercise, you make a circle with your leg.

Begin with your feet together and your hands on your waist. Put your weight on your left foot and, breathing in, lift your right leg straight out in front of you and circle it to the side. Breathing out, circle it to the back and bring it down behind you, allowing your toes to touch the ground. Breathing in, lift your leg up behind you and circle it around to the side. Breathing out, continue the circle to the front, then lower your leg and put your foot on the ground, allowing your weight to again be on both feet. Now do the exercise with the other leg.

Repeat the series of movements three more times.

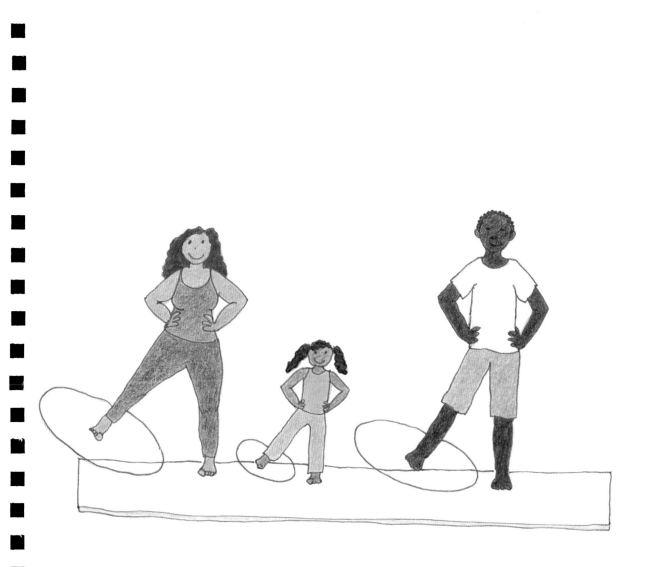

This exercise is done in a lunge position. Begin standing with feet together. Keeping your left foot where it is, move your right foot out so your feet are wider than shoulder-width apart and turn your right foot out 90°. Keeping your weight on both feet, your body will naturally turn slightly toward the right foot to find a comfortable position angled between your two feet. Put your left hand on your waist and your right arm at your side. Breathing in, bend your right knee, bringing your weight over your right foot as you lift your right arm with the palm of your hand facing outward in front of you, and stretch it to the sky! Breathe out, straightening your knee and bringing your right arm back to your side. Repeat the movement three more times.

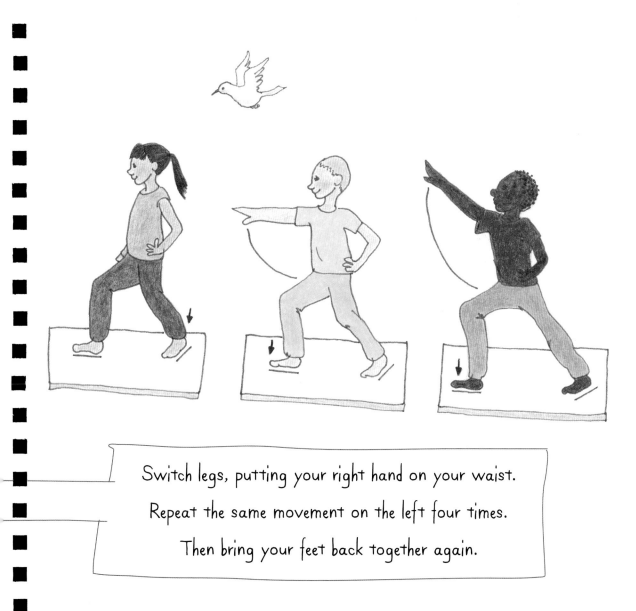

Switch legs, putting your right hand on your waist.

Repeat the same movement on the left four times.

Then bring your feet back together again.

You have finished the Ten Mindful Movements.

Stand firmly on your two feet and breathe in and out. Feel

your body relax.

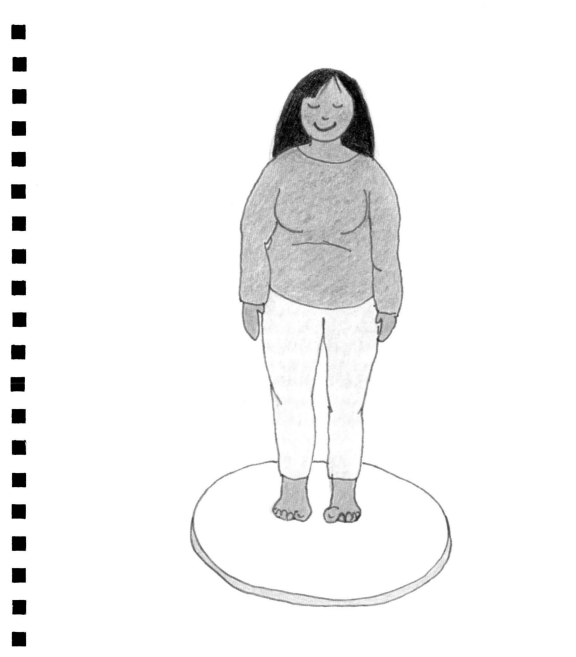

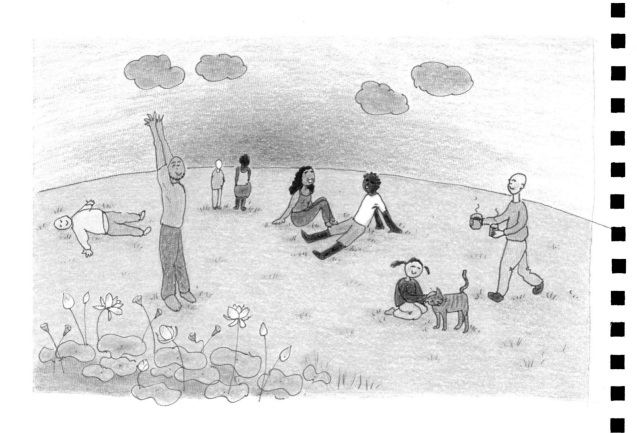

Enjoy your breathing.

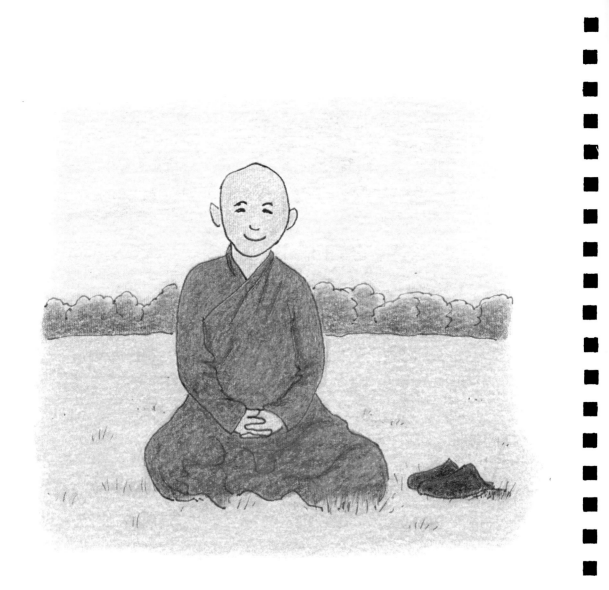

ABOUT THICH NHAT HANH

THICH NHAT HANH was born Nguyen Xuan Bao in Vietnam in 1926. He now lives in southwest France. Along with His Holiness the Dalai Lama, he is considered one of the most influential teachers of Buddhism and a leading spokesperson for the Buddhist peace movement. He is a lifelong advocate for peace, human rights, and social justice.

In all his teachings, Thich Nhat Hanh places a high value on relating ancient wisdom to everyday life. "There is no enlightenment outside of everyday life," says Thich Nhat Hanh. Being present in the moment, he says, is what will bring us happiness. By bringing one's body and mind together in the present moment, we can experience peace and a unity with humanity and with all of life.

At the age of sixteen, Thich Nhat Hanh joined Tu Hieu Zen Monastery near Hue in Central Vietnam, where he began his education as a monk. During the Vietnam War, he worked with others to renew Buddhism and make it more responsive to the needs of society. He felt that if all the Buddhist groups could unify, they could offer an alternative vision of society, one based on the Buddhist principles of compassion and inclusiveness. In 1949, soon after his full ordination, he left Hue to go to Saigon. There he helped found the South Vietnam School of Buddhist Studies. In 1955, he became the editor of *Vietnamese Buddhism,* a journal that was inspirational for young peace activists.

In 1954, Vietnam had been divided and the Diem regime was established in the south. Diem instituted harsh policies against Buddhism. There were nonviolent protests and many monks, nuns, and laypeople were arrested, especially in the early 1960s. In 1963, Nhat Hanh's commitment to nonviolence and his efforts to renew Buddhism brought him an invitation to teach Buddhism at Columbia University in New York.

In 1964, he returned to his home country, to Saigon where he founded the School of Youth for Social Service (SYSS). The SYSS trained young monks, nuns, and laypeople as social workers. They helped rebuild villages and relocate refugees, and provided food, education, medical supplies, and spiritual support for people whose lives had been shattered by the war.

Many SYSS students were attacked and even killed. In 1966, Nhat Hanh helped found the Tiep Hien Order, the Order of Interbeing. The order dedicates itself to the support of Buddhism, mindfulness, social responsibility, and nonviolence. Soon after founding the order, Nhat Hanh traveled to the U.S. to inform people of the effects of the war and to call for peace. He met with officials in the U.S. government and went on an extensive speaking tour of North American cities. It was during this time that he met Dr. Martin Luther King, Jr.

and Thomas Merton. When word of his efforts reached Vietnam, he was refused permission to return home.

After the war, Thich Nhat Hanh continued to travel extensively in Europe and America, sharing his teachings. He hoped to return home after the signing of the 1973 peace agreement that ended the Vietnam War. But the Vietnamese government still considered him an enemy because he would not take sides, and he was forced to remain in exile.

While in Singapore for a conference, Nhat Hanh heard of the plight of the Vietnamese boat people. Singapore, Malaysia, and other countries rejected Vietnamese refugees, who were often pushed back out to sea in ramshackle boats. He helped lead an effort to rescue boat people in the Gulf of Siam and tried to publicize their plight so that countries around the world would raise their refugee quotas.

In 1982, with members of the Order of Interbeing, Thich Nhat Hanh founded Plum Village, a meditation and retreat center near Bordeaux, France, where he still lives today. Monks and nuns from many countries live there together year-round as a Sangha, or spiritual family. Living together, they focus on being the peace they would like to see in the world. The center also welcomes lay practitioners and families, bringing together people from all over the world.

In January 2005, for the first time in thirty-nine years, Thich Nhat Hanh was allowed to return for a three-month visit to Vietnam. He returned for another visit in 2007.

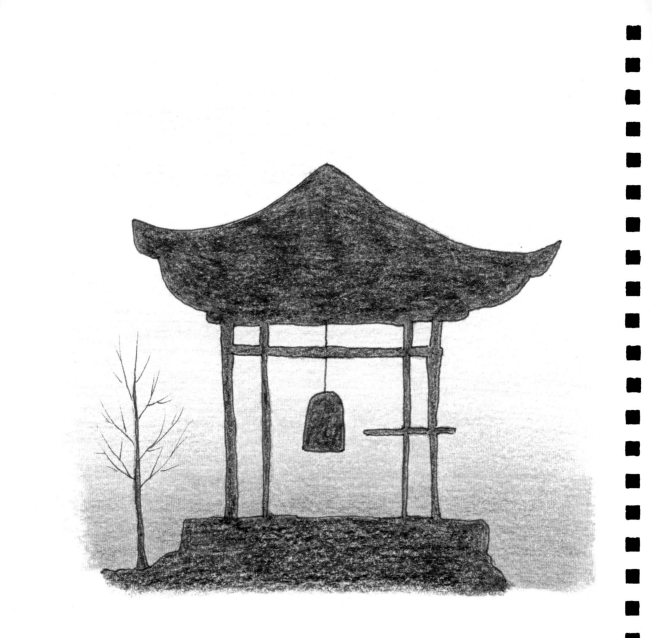

THE VIRTUOUS MAN

The two leaves of the pinewood gate fall shut.
A shimmering arrow leaves the bow,
speeds upward, splits the sky, and explodes the sun.

The blossoms of the orange trees fall
until the courtyard is carpeted—

flickering reflection
of infinity.

Thich Nhat Hanh

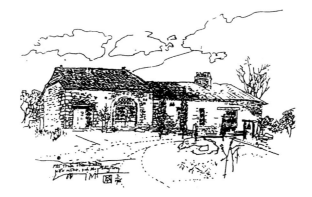

Monastics and laypeople practice the art of mindful living in the tradition of
Thich Nhat Hanh at retreat communities in France and the United States.
To reach any of these communities, or for information about individuals
and families joining for a practice period, please contact:

Plum Village
13 Martineau
33580 Dieulivol, France
www.plumvillage.org

Blue Cliff Monastery
3 Mindfulness Road
Pine Bush, NY 12566
www.bluecliffmonastery.org

Deer Park Monastery
2499 Melru Lane
Escondido, CA 92026
deerpark@plumvillage.org

For a worldwide directory of Sanghas practicing in the tradition
of Thich Nhat Hanh, please visit www.iamhome.org

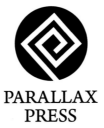

PARALLAX
PRESS

PARALLAX PRESS, a nonprofit organization, publishes books on engaged Buddhism and the practice of mindfulness by Thich Nhat Hanh and other authors. All of Thich Nhat Hanh's work is available at our online store and in our free catalog. For a copy of the catalog, please contact:

Parallax Press
P.O. Box 7355
Berkeley, CA 94707
Tel: (510) 525-0101
www.parallax.org